Chair Yoga for Seniors Over 60

A Comprehensive Guide To Thriving In Your Golden Years With Health, Happiness, And Purpose Under 4 Weeks…

Copyright © [2024] by Dr Alton

Protected by copyright law. No piece of this distribution might be imitated, disseminated, or communicated in any structure or using any and all means, including copying, recording, or other electronic or mechanical techniques, without the earlier composed authorization of the distributer, with the exception of brief citations epitomized in basic surveys and certain other noncommercial purposes allowed by intellectual property regulation.

Table of contents

Contents

Chair Yoga for Seniors Over 60 1

A Comprehensive Guide to Thriving in Your Golden Years with Health, Happiness, and Purpose under 4 weeks... 1

Copyright © [2024] by Dr Alton 2

Table of contents 3

Introduction 5

First Section: Getting Started 9

Part 2: Essential Seat Yoga Postures 13

Section 3: Strategies for Taking In seat..18

Section 4: Seat Yoga Schedule 24

Part 5: Further developing Adaptability and Equilibrium.........30

Part 6: Unwinding and Contemplation 36

Part 6: Unwinding and Contemplation 42

Seventh Segment: Reward Health Tips 48

Section 8: Wellbeing Contemplations 53

Part 9: Regularly Got clarification on some pressing issues 60

Part 10: Final Thoughts: 67

Reward Wellbeing Tips: 72

Introduction

Welcome to the Seat Yoga for Seniors More than 60 Aide, intended to engage and move people in their brilliant years to upgrade their prosperity through the delicate act of yoga. As we age, keeping up with actual adaptability, mental clearness, and close to home equilibrium turns out to be progressively significant. Seat yoga offers a protected and open way for seniors to encounter the various advantages of yoga without the requirement for a yoga mat or confounded presents.

In this aide, we will investigate an assortment of seat based works out, breathing procedures, and contemplation rehearses custom fitted explicitly for seniors. Whether you are a carefully prepared yogi or totally new to the training, this guide plans to give an easy to understand and charming way to deal with integrating yoga into your everyday daily practice.

Why Seat Yoga?

Seat yoga is an amazing choice for seniors, as it permits people with changing degrees of portability and wellness to encounter the groundbreaking impacts of yoga. The training is versatile to various capacities, making it reasonable for the individuals who might experience issues with customary standing or floor-based yoga presents.

- Upgraded Adaptability for seniors north of 60: Increment impact flexibility and joint versatility, in this manner diminishing firmness that is regularly connected with maturing.

- Further developed Balance and Adequacy: support center muscles and added foster equilibrium, reducing the bet of falls.

- Stress decrease: Learn strong loosening up and thought methodology to supervise tension and advance mental thriving.

- Better quieting: Coordinate breath notice to additionally foster lung breaking point and advance respiratory prosperity.

- Neighborhood: interface a neighborhood comparative individuals, gladdening social affiliations and a sensation of having a spot.

Focus on Security Preceding starting your seat yoga venture; focusing on safety is fundamental. Make sure seat yoga is appropriate for your condition by discussing it with your doctor. Persistently focus on your body and change rehearses dependent upon the situation. This guide is planned to enhance, not replace, capable clinical insight.

By and by, we ought to leave on a trip of dealing with oneself and centrality through the demonstration of Seat Yoga for Seniors More than 60. Plan to embrace the interminable physical, mental, and significant benefits that this accessible sort of yoga offers of real value!

First Section: Getting Started

Chair yoga is the first exciting step toward better health and vitality. In order to ensure that your seat yoga experience is pleasant and agreeable, we'll walk you through the fundamental steps in this section.

Choosing the Right Seat Choosing the right seat is essential for a successful seat yoga practice. Choose a consistent seat with a straight back and no wheels. To prevent accidental tipping, make sure the seat is on a level surface. The seat should allow you to sit with your feet level on the ground, molding a 90-degree point at your knees.

Wearing Garments That Are Agreeable

Placed on garments that are not difficult to move in and that are free and agreeable. This will promise you can totally take part in the seat yoga gives no limits. Consider breathable surfaces that grant your skin to stay cool during the preparation.

Making a Serene Shelter Make a devoted space for your seat yoga practice. Pick a peaceful locale where you will not be quickly vexed. Clear the space of any typical obstructions to guarantee a protected practice. During your workout, having a bottle of water close by can also help you stay hydrated.

Spreading out Care Require several seconds to concentrate yourself before beginning your seat yoga practice. Relax in your chair, close your eyes, and inhale deeply. License your mid-area to reach out as you take in significantly through your nose and inhale out relaxed through your mouth. This immediate thought practice assists you with progressing into the continuous second, setting up your psyche and body for the arrangement ahead.

Seat Game-plan

Position your seat looking forward, guaranteeing that there is adequate room around you to straightforwardly move your arms and legs. If you're watching a video or reading a book, make sure your screen or instructor can be seen clearly from your seated position.

Adjustments and Props If that you truly have any desire to, you ought to use props like cushions or blocks to make your preparation more pleasant. Be prepared to adapt to meet your particular requirements as well. Each body is surprising, and arrange yoga can be changed as per oblige different cutoff points and constraints.

As you emerge as alright with these significant contemplations, you're prepared to jump into the universe of seat yoga. We'll look at delicate postures, breathing techniques, and loosening exercises specifically designed for seniors over 60 in the going with areas. Plan to partake in the potential gains of seat yoga at your own speed!

Part 2: Essential Seat Yoga Postures

Now that you've made way for your seat yoga practice, we should investigate a few essential represents that advance adaptability, versatility, and unwinding. A delightful introduction to chair yoga is provided by these easy movements, which are intended for seniors over 60.

1. Neck Stretches

- *Sit serenely on your seat with your spine straight.
- *Breathe in, stretching your spine, and as you breathe out, tenderly slant your head aside, bringing your ear towards your shoulder.

- *Hold the stretch for a couple of breaths, feeling the delicate stretch at the edge of your neck.
- *Rehash on the opposite side.

2. Shoulder Rolls

- *Sit tall and loosen up your arms by your sides.
- *Breathe in as you lift your shoulders towards your ears.
- *Breathe out and move your shoulders back and down in a round movement.
- *Rehash for a few rounds, then switch headings.

- *Sit with your spine straight and feet level on the ground.
- *Breathe in to protract your spine, and as you breathe out, contort your middle aside.
- *Clutch the rear of the seat for help and investigate your shoulder.
- *Hold for a couple of breaths, then, at that point, rehash on the opposite side.

3. Delicate Situated Ahead Twists

1. *Sit with your feet level on the ground, hip-width separated.
2. *Breathe in and extend your spine, then breathe out as you pivot at your hips and incline forward.

3. *Arrive at your hands towards the floor or handle the sides of the seat.
4. *Hold the stretch for a couple of breaths, feeling the delivery in your lower back and hamstrings.

4. *Sit comfortably with your feet flat on the ground for the ankle circles.

- *Start circling your ankle in the clockwise direction by lifting one foot slightly off the ground.
- *After a couple of pivots, change to counterclockwise.
- *Rehash with the other lower leg.

5. Wrist Activities

- *Broaden your arms before you at shoulder level.
- *Flex and broaden your wrists, moving your hands all over.
- *Turn your wrists clockwise and afterward counterclockwise.
- *This aids in enhancing wrist and forearm mobility.

These fundamental seat yoga presents give an establishment to your training. Make sure to move gradually, and assuming that any posture feels awkward, make changes in accordance with suit your solace level. In the following part, we'll investigate breathing methods to supplement your actual practice and upgrade in general prosperity.

Section 3: Strategies for Taking In seat

Yoga, merging turn of events and breathing is a crucial part that updates the real practice as well as engages mental clearness and loosening up. In this section, we'll look at seat-based breathing techniques that are easy to incorporate into your daily schedule and are clear and convincing.

1. *Sit happily with a as the crow flies spine to unwind the diaphragm.

- *Put one pass on your upper body and the other resting on your midsection.
- *Take a full breath in through your nose and let your waist broaden.

- *Breathe in out agreeable through your mouth, feeling your mid-district contract.
- *Base on breathing fundamentally into your stomach, advancing relaxing.

2. Sea Breath (Ujjayi Pranayama)

- *Sit tall and take a full breath in through your nose.
- *Breathe in out agreeable through somewhat contracted throat, making a delicate "sea like" sound.
- *Take in and inhale out with this sensitive sound, permitting it to coordinate your breathing velocity.
- *Ujjayi breathing helps you with focusing in on your breath and calms your mind.

3. Substitute nasal breathing (Nadi Shodhana)

- *Sit comfortably and relax your left leg close to your left knee.
- *Utilizing your right hand, pass your summary and spotlight fingers on to rest between your eyebrows.
- *Take in through your left nostril and close your right nostril with your thumb.
- *Close your left nostril with your ring finger, discharge the right nostril, and breathe in out.
- *Take in through the right nostril, close it, discharge the left nostril, and breathe in out.
- *This planning helps balance the development of energy in the body.

4. Box Unwinding *Comfortably inhale up to the number four.

- *Stop your unwinding for a count of four.
- *Breathe in out agreeable to a count of four.
- *Stop for an incorporate of four going prior to taking in once more.
- *Rehash this cycle for several rounds, changing the consider wonderful.

5. Stunning Loosening up

1. *Sit successfully and shut your eyes.
2. *Take in through your nose for a count of four.

3. *For a count of six, inhale through your mouth.
4. *Rotate around the sound and beat of your breath.
5. *Blasting breathing instigates a condition of quietness and relaxing.

Integrating Breath Into Positions During your seat yoga practice, synchronize your movements with your breath. Take in when a stance is stretching or opening, and exhale when it is narrowing or conveying. This coordination further fosters the frontal cortex body connection, moving a vibe of transfer and care in your planning.

We will look at a typical seat yoga routine that combines these postures with breathing exercises to give you an all-encompassing experience in the following section.

Section 4: Seat Yoga Schedule

Now that you've gotten comfortable with fundamental seat yoga postures and breathing methods, now is the ideal time to assemble them into an amicable daily practice. This part will direct you through an example seat yoga grouping planned explicitly for seniors north of 60. This normal expects to upgrade adaptability, further develop balance, and develop a feeling of unwinding.

Warm-Up: Diaphragmatic Relaxing

Sit easily in your seat with a straight spine.

Put single hand on your upper body and the additional on your midsection.

Respire in intensely through your nose, permit your midsection to extend.

Using your mouth, slowly exhale while feeling your abdomen contract.

Perform diaphragmatic relaxing for 2-3 minutes to focus and get ready for the training.

Pose 1: Neck Stretches

Breathe in, protract your spine, and breathe out as you tenderly slant your head aside.

Hold for a couple of breaths, feeling the stretch at the edge of your neck.

Rehash on the opposite side.

Perform 2 sets on each side.

Pose 2: Shoulder Rolls:

Take a deep breath in as you raise your shoulders to the ears.

Breathe out and move your shoulders back and down in a roundabout movement.

Rehash for 1 moment, exchanging bearings partially through.

Pose 3: Situated Turns

Breathe in to stretch your spine, breathe out as you curve your middle aside.

While looking over your shoulder, hold on to the chair's back for support.

Continue on the opposite side after holding for thirty seconds.

Pose 4: Delicate Situated Ahead Curve

Breathe in and extend your spine, breathe out as you pivot at your hips and incline forward.

Hold for 30 seconds, feeling the delivery in your lower back and hamstrings.

Pose 5: Lower leg Circles

Lift one foot somewhat off the floor and circle your lower leg clockwise.

Change to counterclockwise after a couple of pivots.

Rehash with the other lower leg.

Perform 1 moment for every lower leg.

Pose 6: Wrist Activities

Broaden your arms before you at shoulder level.

Flex and expand your wrists, moving your hands all over.

Perform a clockwise and then a counterclockwise wrist rotation.

Perform for 1 moment.

Breathing Reconciliation

Breathe in during the protracting period of each posture and breathe out during the compression or delivering stage.

Practice Sea Breath (Ujjayi Pranayama) during situated presents.

Cool Down: Unwinding Posture

Sit serenely, shut your eyes, and spotlight on your breath.

Take a profound gasp in, breathe out fully, and let your remains relax.

Burn through 3-5 minutes in this unwinding present.

Congrats on finishing your seat yoga schedule! Go ahead and rehash this succession consistently, step by step expanding the span or power as you become more alright with the postures. In the following part, we'll investigate ways of upgrading your adaptability and equilibrium through extra stretches and works out.

Part 5: Further developing Adaptability and Equilibrium

In this part, we'll dive further into seat yoga represents that explicitly target adaptability and equilibrium. These activities are intended to upgrade joint versatility, further develop muscle adaptability, and reinforce center muscles, adding to a general feeling of prosperity. Make sure to pay attention to your body and progress at your own speed.

Pose 1: Leg raises from a seated position Relax and place your feet flat on the ground.

Breathe in, extend your spine, and breathe out as you lift one leg straight before you.

Hold for a couple of breaths, flexing your foot for added stretch.

On the other side, lower the leg and repeat.

Do two sets for each leg.

Pose 2: Situated Side Stretch

Sit with your feet level on the ground, hip-width separated.

Take a cavernous gasp along by raise your arms above your head.

Breathe out and incline tenderly aside, feeling a stretch along your middle.

Continue on the opposite side after holding for thirty seconds.

Perform 2 sets on each side.

Pose 3: Situated Knee Embrace

Sit tall and expand one leg straight out.

Breathe in, lift the knee of your other leg towards your chest, embracing it with two hands.

Hold for 30 seconds, feeling a stretch in your hip and lower back.

Rehash on the opposite side.

Perform 2 sets on each side.

Pose 4: Situated Figure-Four Stretch

Sit tall with your feet level on the ground.

Get one lower leg over the contrary knee, making a figure-four shape.

Breathe in and sit up tall, breathe out and tenderly push on the crossed knee, feeling a stretch in your hip.

Continue on the opposite side after holding for thirty seconds.

Perform 2 sets on each side.

Pose 5: Situated Tree Posture

Sit with your spine straight and feet level on the ground.

Lift one foot and spot the underside against the internal thigh of the contrary leg.

Track down your equilibrium and hold for 30 seconds.

Rehash on the opposite side.

Perform 2 sets on each side.

Pose 6: Stretch like a seated cat or cow Lie down with your hands on your knees.

Breathe in as you curve your back, lifting your chest (Cow).

Breathe out as you round your spine, tucking your jaw to your chest (Feline).

Stream between these two situations for 1 moment.

Integration of Balance When performing balance poses, keep your eyes fixed on a single point to stabilize your posture.

Utilize the seat for help if necessary, progressively depending on it less as your equilibrium moves along.

Cool Down: Relaxation Pose: Perform the Relaxation Pose from Chapter 4 at the end of your session to let your body absorb the benefits of your practice.

Consistently integrating these adaptability and equilibrium centered presents into your normal will add to expanded portability and security over the long haul. In the following section, we'll investigate unwinding and reflection strategies to additional improve your general prosperity.

Part 6: Unwinding and Contemplation

In this section, we'll investigate unwinding and reflection strategies intended to quiet the brain, lessen pressure, and improve your general feeling of prosperity. These practices are vital to seat yoga for seniors, giving a comprehensive way to deal with wellbeing.

Unwinding Posture

Savasana (Carcass Posture):

Sit easily with your eyes shut.

take breaths in intensely through your nose and take breaths out entirely through your oral cavity.

allow your cadaver to unwind, beginning from your toes and stirring up to your top.

Remain in this casual state for 5-10 minutes, zeroing in on your breath.

Directed Reflection

Careful Breathing Reflection:

Sit easily, zeroing in on your breath.

Breathe in profoundly, building up to four, and breathe out leisurely to the count of six.

As considerations emerge, recognize them without judgment and delicately take your concentration back to your breath.

Spend ten minutes practicing.

Body Output Reflection:

Shut your eyes and focus on various pieces of your body, beginning from your toes.

Notice any strain or sensations, and intentionally discharge pressure as you travel through each body part.

Progress from your toes to the highest point of your head.

Practice for 10-15 minutes.

Seat Yoga Nidra

Yoga Nidra (Yogic Rest):

Sit serenely with eyes shut, paying attention to a directed Yoga Nidra contemplation.

To bring awareness to various parts of your body, emotions, and breath, follow the instructions.

Experience a secret government of unwinding, advancing mental lucidity and inward harmony.

Practice for 20-30 minutes.

Walking mindfully Walking mindfully:

In the event that conceivable, stand up and clutch the rear of the seat for help.

Take slow, purposeful advances, zeroing in on the vibe of each foot lifting and contacting the ground.

Practice for 5-10 minutes.

Appreciation Reflection

Appreciation Reflection:

Sit serenely and consider three things you're appreciative for.

Shut your eyes and picture every one of these things, feeling a feeling of appreciation.

Practice for 5-10 minutes.

Integration into Daily Life Include brief meditation breaks into your daily routine to cultivate mindfulness and focus on your breath.

Utilize directed reflection applications or accounts to investigate different contemplation styles.

Normal act of these unwinding and contemplation strategies will add to a more noteworthy feeling of internal harmony and profound prosperity. We'll look at bonus health advice in the next chapter, including how to eat right, stay hydrated, and do low-impact exercises to lose weight.

Part 6: Unwinding and Contemplation

In this section, we'll investigate unwinding and reflection strategies intended to quiet the brain, lessen pressure, and improve your general feeling of prosperity. These practices are vital to seat yoga for seniors, giving a comprehensive way to deal with wellbeing.

Unwinding Posture

Savasana (Carcass Posture):

Sit easily with your eyes shut.

respire in deeply through your beak and breathe out completely from beginning to end your mouth.

Permit your body to slow down, start as of your toes and stirring awake to your head.

Remain in this casual state for 5-10 minutes, zeroing in on your breath.

Directed Reflection

Careful Breathing Reflection:

Sit easily, zeroing in on your breath.

Breathe in profoundly, building up to four, and breathe out leisurely to the count of six.

As considerations emerge, recognize them without judgment and delicately take your concentration back to your breath.

Spend ten minutes practicing.

Body Output Reflection:

Shut your eyes and focus on various pieces of your body, beginning from your toes.

Notice any strain or sensations, and intentionally discharge pressure as you travel through each body part.

Progress from your toes to the highest point of your head.

Practice for 10-15 minutes.

Seat Yoga Nidra

Yoga Nidra (Yogic Rest):

Sit serenely with eyes shut, paying attention to a directed Yoga Nidra contemplation.

To bring awareness to various parts of your body, emotions, and breath, follow the instructions.

Experience a secret government of unwinding, advancing mental lucidity and inward harmony.

Practice for 20-30 minutes.

Walking mindfully

Walking mindfully:

In the event that conceivable, stand up and clutch the rear of the seat for help.

Take slow, purposeful advances, zeroing in on the vibe of each foot lifting and contacting the ground.

Practice for 5-10 minutes.

Appreciation Reflection

Appreciation Reflection:

Sit serenely and consider three things you're appreciative for.

Shut your eyes and picture every one of these things, feeling a feeling of appreciation.

Practice for 5-10 minutes.

Integration into Daily Life Include brief meditation breaks into your daily routine to cultivate mindfulness and focus on your breath.

Utilize directed reflection applications or accounts to investigate different contemplation styles.

Normal act of these unwinding and contemplation strategies will add to a more noteworthy feeling of internal harmony and profound prosperity. We'll look at bonus health advice in the next chapter, including how to eat right, stay hydrated, and do low-impact exercises to lose weight.

Seventh Segment: Reward Health Tips

In this part, we will take a gander at extra health tips that you can use to enhance your seat yoga practice and further develop your general prosperity. For weighting the board, these ideas cover hydration, nourishment, and integrating low-influence rehearses.

Tip 1: Advice for Seniors on How to Eat a Healthy, Adapted Diet: Your essential spotlight ought to be on a careful nutritional plan that is even and incorporates various natural products, vegetables, lean proteins, entire grains, dairy or dairy choices.

Control of Section: By being aware of the sizes of the pieces, you can maintain a solid weight during backing processing.

Vitamin D and calcium: Guarantee a tasteful affirmation of calcium and vitamin D for bone thriving, either through dietary sources or upgrades as proposed by your clinical thought supplier.

Hydration: To keep hydrated and support generally wellbeing, hydrate over the course of the day.

Tip 2: To remain hydrated, drinking sufficient water is significant: Plan to drink something like 8 glasses (64 ounces) of water consistently, changing considering your specific necessities and advancement level.

Hydration Advantages: Genuine hydration keeps up with assimilation, joint success, and generally real cycles.

Normal Teas: For grouping and additional hydration benefits, integrate normal teas or blended water.

Tip 3: Organizing Low-Effect Activities for Weight decline

Strolling: Take regular, low-impact steps like walking. Go all shortly out of each and every day, multiple times consistently.

Swimming: Consider water aerobics or swimming, which provide a full-body workout with minimal joint impact.

Seat Activities: To increment calorie utilization, supplement your seat yoga routine with extra low-influence exercises like leg lifts or situated strolls.

Tip 4: Schedule for Quality Rest and Unwinding: Spread out a predictable rest plan, going for the stars critical length of huge worth rest every evening.

Rest Climate: Create an environment that is peaceful and comfortable for sleeping with a sturdy sleeping pad and cushion.

Evening Plan: Spread out a peaceful regular practice for the evening and go without partaking in animating activities before rest time.

Attempt to speak with your clinical advantages supplier going before doing essential improvements to your eating routine or work-out normal practice, particularly tolerating you have any basic diseases.

In the going with region, we'll address security assessments, average thriving burdens for seniors, and the significance of chatting with clinical advantages experts going before start or changing any development or flourishing related program.

Section 8: Wellbeing Contemplations

Guaranteeing your wellbeing is central while taking part in any activity or wellbeing related exercises, particularly as a senior. This part will address normal security contemplations, give direction on adjusting activities to explicit circumstances, and accentuate the significance of talking with medical care experts.

Normal Wellbeing Worries for Seniors

Heart Conditions:

Joint inflammation and Joint Issues:

Pick seat yoga stances and activities that are delicate on the joints.

Pay attention to your body, and keep away from developments that cause agony or distress.

Osteoporosis:

Integrate weight-bearing activities into your everyday practice to help bone wellbeing.

If you have osteoporosis, avoid forward bends and twists.

Balance Concerns:

Utilize the seat or other stable surfaces for help during balance works out.

Perform balance practices close to a wall or durable household item for added security.

Diabetes:

Screen glucose levels, particularly assuming participating in exercises that might affect glucose levels.

Remain hydrated and have a tidbit if necessary.

Adjusting Activities for Explicit Circumstances

Hypertension:

Abstain from pausing your breathing during works out; all things considered, center around consistent and controlled relaxing.

Alter represents that include abrupt changes ready.

Back Pain:

Pick delicate stretches that give alleviation without causing strain.

Counsel a medical services proficient for custom fitted activities that address your particular condition.

Restricted Versatility:

Alter stances to oblige your scope of movement.

Continuously progress to further developed acts like your adaptability moves along.

Mental Wellbeing:

Practice care reflection to help mental prosperity.

Assuming memory concerns emerge, consider integrating mental activities into your daily schedule.

Counsel with Medical care Experts

Prior to Beginning a Program:

Get leeway from your medical services supplier prior to starting any activity or wellbeing related program.

Share your advantage in seat yoga and talk about any current wellbeing concerns or restrictions.

Standard Registrations:

Keep your medical care supplier informed about your advancement and any progressions in your wellbeing.

Talk about changes or acclimations to your routine in light of their suggestions.

Advice from a professional:

Think about consulting a physical therapist or fitness professional who specializes in working with seniors.

They can offer you exercises and guidance that are specific to your needs.

You'll be better able to take advantage of chair yoga and other health-related activities if you place safety first and seek professional guidance. In the following section, we'll resolve every now and again posed inquiries about seat yoga for seniors.

Part 9: Regularly Got clarification on some pressing issues

This part tends to normal questions and worries that seniors might have about seat yoga. Understanding these habitually posed inquiries can assist with upgrading your certainty and happiness as you set out on your seat yoga venture.

1. Is seat yoga reasonable for all wellness levels?

Indeed, seat yoga is profoundly versatile and can be adjusted to suit different wellness levels. Whether you are a fledgling or have some involvement in yoga, seat yoga gives a delicate and open method for receiving the rewards of yoga practice.

2. Might I at any point actually rehearse seat yoga on the off chance that I have restricted versatility?

Absolutely! Seat yoga is explicitly intended to oblige people with restricted versatility. Many postures can be adjusted to various scopes of movement, guaranteeing that you can serenely take an interest and experience the constructive outcomes of the training.

3. How frequently would it be advisable for me to rehearse seat yoga?

The recurrence of your seat yoga practice relies upon your singular inclinations and state of being. Beginning with a couple of meetings each week and steadily expanding recurrence is a decent methodology. Consistency is critical, so go for the gold that you can reasonably keep up with.

4. Is chair yoga a good way to manage pain?

Indeed, seat yoga can be helpful for overseeing torment, particularly in conditions like joint pain or constant back torment. Notwithstanding, it's pivotal to stand by listening to your body, stay away from places that cause uneasiness, and talk with your medical care supplier assuming you have explicit worries about torment the board.

5. Can chair yoga alleviate anxiety and stress?

Certainly. Seat yoga consolidates care and unwinding procedures, making it a compelling device for overseeing pressure and uneasiness. Meditation, gentle movements, and concentrating on the breath all contribute to a sense of calm and mental well-being.

6. How long ought to each seat yoga meeting last?

The span of your seat yoga meeting can shift in view of your inclinations and timetable. A meeting can go from 15 to 30 minutes or longer, contingent upon the time you have accessible. Zeroing in on consistency than on the length of every session is more significant.

7. Can chair yoga help me sleep better?

Indeed, the unwinding and care parts of seat yoga can add to further developed rest quality. Laying out a predictable sleep time schedule that incorporates seat yoga unwinding postures can help sign to your body that now is the right time to slow down.

8. Are there explicit seat yoga models for explicit medical issue?

Indeed, seat yoga stances can be adjusted to address explicit medical issue. In the event that you have worries about a specific condition, consider talking with a medical services supplier or a certified yoga educator who can fit stances to your singular requirements.

9. Is it necessary to speak with a doctor before beginning chair yoga?

Indeed, it's fitting to talk with your medical services supplier prior to beginning any new activity program, including seat yoga. Based on your health history, they can offer insight into any particular considerations or adjustments you may require.

10. Could seat yoga be a social action?

Absolutely. Seat yoga classes or gathering meetings give a social and steady climate. Joining a class can offer the valuable chance to interface with others, share encounters, and cultivate a feeling of local area.

In the last part, we'll wrap up the aide with an end, summing up key important points and empowering you to proceed with your seat yoga practice for supported prosperity.

Part 10: Final Thoughts:

Thank you so much for finishing the Chair Yoga for Seniors Over 60 Guide! This excursion has furnished you with the instruments and information to set out on a satisfying seat yoga practice customized to your requirements and inclinations. Let's go over some important takeaways and encourage you to keep going down this well-being path.

Key Focus points:

Adaptability: Seat yoga is profoundly versatile, making it reasonable for people of all wellness levels and capacities. The training can be customized to address explicit wellbeing concerns and constraints.

Consistency is Vital: Laying out a steady seat yoga routine is a higher priority than the span of every meeting. Customary practice adds to further developed adaptability, equilibrium, and by and large prosperity.

Connection Between the Mind and the Body: Seat yoga accentuates the psyche body association through the joining of breath, development, and care. This all encompassing methodology upholds actual wellbeing as well as mental and close to home prosperity.

Security First: Focus on wellbeing by picking represents that line up with your capacities and talking with medical services experts prior to beginning any new activity program.

Local area and Social Association: Seat yoga can be a social movement, giving chances to join classes or gathering meetings, cultivating associations with others on a comparative health venture.

Hydration and nourishment: A well-balanced diet, adequate hydration, and healthy lifestyle choices can help your chair yoga practice.

Meeting with Medical Professionals: Routinely speak with your medical care supplier, refreshing them on your seat yoga practice and tending to any wellbeing concerns or changes.

Last Thoughts of Encouragement:

As you proceed with your seat yoga venture, recollect that progress is a steady interaction. Celebrate little accomplishments, remain aware of your body's necessities, and partake in the feeling of prosperity that accompanies standard practice.

Investigate extra assets, go to seat yoga classes, or associate with nearby networks to improve your experience. Seat yoga is a flexible and pleasant method for keeping up with and work on your wellbeing, giving both physical and mental advantages.

Much thanks to you for going along with us on this excursion toward improved prosperity through Seat Yoga for Seniors North of 60. May your way be overflowing with satisfaction, imperativeness, and a profound association with your own wellbeing and bliss. Enjoy your practice!

Reward Wellbeing Tips:

Tip 1: Nourishment for Seniors

Stress a decent eating routine with lean proteins, organic products, vegetables, and entire grains.

Consider counseling a nutritionist for customized guidance.

Tip 2: Hydration

Hydrate over the course of the day to help generally wellbeing and prosperity.

Tip 3: Low-Effect Exercise for Weight reduction

Join seat yoga with low-influence practices like strolling or swimming for powerful weight the board.

Counsel a wellness proficient for a custom-made practice plan.

Tip 4: Quality Rest

Focus on great rest cleanliness, including a predictable rest plan and an agreeable rest climate.

Keep in mind, it's generally prudent for seniors to talk with their medical services suppliers prior to beginning another activity or health improvement plan.